HEAL YOUR PAST

Let Go of Emotional Wounds, Restore Peace of Mind, Build Unbreakable Confidence, and Turn Trauma into Your Greatest Strength

Dr. Maureen Tigga

ABOUT THE AUTHOR

Dr. Maureen Tigga, Author of "Heal Your Past."

Dr. Maureen Tigga is an accomplished gynecologist with over 15 years of clinical experience. Writing has always been her passion, and she has numerous publications in various prestigious medical journals. Recently, Dr. Tigga has expanded her focus to authoring books, bringing her extensive knowledge to a new series on women's mental health.Throughout her career, she has actively taken part in several research projects and studies, earning accolades for her contributions to the field of gynecology. Dr. Tigga is a proud member of the Royal College of Obstetricians and Gynecologists, London, a testament to her dedication to excellence in her profession. Additionally, she is a credentialed practitioner with the Indian Menopause Society, reflecting her special interest in menopause medicine. With her vast clinical experience, Dr. Tigga is now committed to addressing the critical and often overlooked aspects of women's mental health through her writing.

ACKNOWLEDGMENTS

I would like to express my gratitude to everyone who has supported me throughout this journey. To my patients, whose stories and experiences have been a constant source of inspiration—thank you for trusting me with your care and for teaching me. Special thanks to my family and friends for their unswerving support and faith in me. Last, to all the women who are traversing this journey called life, this book is for you. Your courage and resilience are the true driving forces behind this work.

DEDICATION

This book is dedicated to all women—To their strength, resilience, and the unspoken battles. May this book serve as a source of understanding, support, and empowerment for every woman who reads it.

CONTENTS

Introduction: Embrace Healing for a Powerful Transformation

"Healing takes courage, and we all have courage, even if we have to dig a little to find it." – Tori Amos

Introduction

Every person carries scars—some visible, many hidden. While physical wounds are easily recognized, emotional wounds often linger beneath the surface, affecting our thoughts, behaviors, and relationships. These unresolved emotional pains, often stemming from trauma, grief, or betrayal, can shape our self-worth, guide our decisions, and block personal growth.

Healing from emotional wounds is not just about moving on from the past. It's about reclaiming control, releasing the grip of painful memories, and creating space for peace, confidence, and happiness. When left unchecked, these wounds fester, subtly guiding how we perceive ourselves and others. Yet, by consciously healing, we open ourselves to a powerful transformation—one that allows us to turn past trauma into a source of strength.

Why Healing the Past Matters

We often hear the phrase, "time heals all wounds." But time alone isn't always enough. Healing is an active process that requires understanding, courage, and intention. Emotional wounds that remain untreated manifest in various ways: anxiety, trust issues, self-sabotage, and even physical symptoms like fatigue and headaches. The longer these wounds are ignored, the deeper their roots grow in our psyche.

Case Study 1: Sarah's Silent Struggle

Sarah was in her mid-30s, a successful marketing manager, and outwardly appeared to have her life together. However, beneath her composed exterior, she carried the emotional scars of a volatile childhood. Raised in a household where anger and emotional neglect were prevalent, Sarah grew up feeling unworthy of love. As an adult, this deeply embedded belief dictated her relationships. She was drawn to partners who were emotionally unavailable, perpetuating a cycle of rejection and hurt.

Sarah's turning point came during a conversation with a close friend, who pointed out a recurring pattern in her relationships. After months of reflection, Sarah began therapy, where she realized that her subconscious belief of being unworthy stemmed from her unresolved childhood wounds. She had unknowingly been seeking validation from others to fill that void. Through therapy and self-awareness, Sarah was able to confront her past, recognize her inherent worth, and gradually let go of the need for external approval.

Breaking Free from Emotional Chains

Emotional wounds act as chains, keeping us bound to the pain of the past. This entrapment often leads to unhealthy coping mechanisms, such as avoidance, denial, or excessive people-pleasing. However, it's possible to break these chains by addressing the root cause of the pain and actively working toward healing.

One effective strategy is cognitive reframing, a technique supported by research in psychology. **Cognitive reframing helps individuals change their interpretation of past events by shifting negative perceptions into more neutral or positive ones.** For example, instead of internalizing a past failure as proof of inadequacy, cognitive reframing encourages seeing it as a learning opportunity.

Scientific Research: A study conducted by Harvard University found that individuals who engage in therapeutic techniques such as cognitive reframing showed significant improvements in emotional resilience and mental well-being. By reshaping their perspective, participants experienced reduced symptoms of depression and anxiety and developed a more balanced self-view (Kross et al., 2020).

Case Study 2: Emma's Journey to Forgiveness

Emma was in her late 20s when she began experiencing severe panic attacks. After multiple visits to doctors and tests ruling out physical causes, she was advised to consult a therapist. Through her therapy sessions, Emma realized that her anxiety was deeply rooted in unresolved trauma from her teenage years when she had experienced a traumatic incident of betrayal by a close friend.

Emma had buried the pain for over a decade, but it had been silently influencing her ability to trust others, particularly in friendships. Through a combination of therapy, journaling, and mindfulness practices, Emma began the process of forgiveness—not just toward the friend who had hurt her, but also toward herself. She learned that holding onto the bitterness and distrust had only perpetuated her anxiety and feelings of isolation. Forgiveness allowed her to release the emotional chains that had kept her in a state of hyper-vigilance, and over time, her panic attacks subsided.

The Journey Ahead: Turning Wounds into Wisdom

Healing is not an overnight process. It is a journey that involves self-reflection, patience, and often professional support. The key lies in transforming emotional wounds into sources of wisdom rather than allowing them to define who we are. This transformation requires reframing trauma and recognizing that we are not our pain—we are the people who survived it.

Cultivating Self-Compassion: Self-compassion plays a pivotal role in the healing process. According to Dr. Kristin Neff, a leading researcher in self-compassion, individuals who practice self-compassion are more resilient in the face of setbacks and experience greater emotional well-being. Self-compassion involves treating oneself with the same kindness and understanding that one would offer to a close friend.

Practical Steps to Turn Pain into Strength:

1. **Acknowledge the Wound**: Denying pain only deepens it. Acknowledgment is the first step toward healing.

2. **Seek Support**: Whether through therapy, support groups, or trusted friends, healing is more effective when we allow others to help us navigate our emotions.

3. **Reframe the Narrative**: Instead of viewing your past as a source of weakness, see it as a chapter in your growth story. Every experience teaches a lesson.

4. **Practice Mindfulness**: Mindfulness techniques, such as meditation and breathing exercises, help ground us in the present moment and reduce emotional overwhelm. A study by the American Psychological Association (APA) highlights the effectiveness of mindfulness in managing stress and

fostering emotional regulation (Grossman et al., 2018).

5. **Celebrate Small Victories**: Healing happens in stages. Celebrate the small steps along the way, whether it's overcoming a negative thought pattern or successfully confronting a difficult memory.

Scientific Research: Research from Stanford University underscores the importance of narrative reframing in healing from trauma. The study shows that individuals who actively engage in rewriting their personal narratives and viewing themselves as survivors, rather than victims, experience increased psychological resilience and a more empowered outlook on life (Pennebaker & Seagal, 2017).

Conclusion

Healing emotional wounds requires courage, time, and commitment. By acknowledging the pain of the past, breaking free from the emotional chains that hold us back, and embracing the wisdom our experiences offer, we can transform trauma into strength. This process enables us to restore peace of mind, build unshakable confidence, and lead lives no longer defined by past wounds but by the strength we've gained from overcoming them.

Sarah and Emma's stories remind us that healing is not linear, but it is possible. It's about taking one step at a time, being patient with oneself, and recognizing that every step forward—no matter how small—is a victory. The journey ahead is one of profound transformation, where emotional wounds become lessons, and trauma becomes a testament to resilience.

Resources

- **Books:**

    a. Neff, K. (2011). *Self-Compassion: The Proven Power of Being Kind to Yourself.* William Morrow Paperbacks.

    b. van der Kolk, B. (2014). *The Body Keeps the Score: Brain, Mind, and Body in the Healing of Trauma.* Viking.

- **Scientific Articles:**

    a. Kross, E., et al. (2020). *Cognitive Reappraisal in Emotional Regulation: How It Works and Why It Matters.* Harvard University.

    b. Grossman, P., et al. (2018). *Mindfulness Practice*

and Its Impact on Emotional Resilience. American Psychological Association.

c. Pennebaker, J.W., & Seagal, J.D. (2017). *The Healing Power of Expressive Writing: Rewriting Trauma Narratives for Psychological Growth.* Stanford University.

- **Therapy and Support:**

  a. *BetterHelp* - Online counseling platform for accessible therapy.

  b. *National Institute for the Clinical Application of Behavioral Medicine (NICABM)* – Resources on mindfulness, self-compassion, and trauma healing techniques.

- **Mindfulness and Meditation:**

  a. *Headspace* - Mindfulness and meditation app to support emotional balance.

  b. *Insight Timer* - Meditation app offering practices tailored to emotional healing.

1

Understanding Emotional Wounds and Their Impact

"The wound is the place where the light enters you." – Rumi

Introduction

Every individual experiences emotional pain at some point in their life. Whether it's the result of a difficult childhood, the loss of a loved one, a broken relationship, or a traumatic experience, emotional wounds cut deep, often leaving lasting impressions that linger for years. Unlike physical wounds, which may heal with time and treatment, emotional wounds tend to hide beneath the surface, shaping our thoughts, perceptions, and behaviors without us even realizing it.

Emotional wounds can be debilitating, silently influencing our self-esteem, confidence, and ability to form healthy relationships. If left unaddressed, they can create negative patterns that repeat throughout our lives, keeping us stuck in cycles of pain, doubt, and emotional instability. In this chapter, we'll explore what emotional wounds are, how they form, and the profound impact they can have on our mental and emotional health.

1. What Are Emotional Wounds?

Emotional wounds are the psychological scars left behind by painful or traumatic experiences. Just like physical wounds, they can vary in severity—from minor disappointments to deep trauma caused by significant life events. These emotional wounds are typically the result of negative experiences such as betrayal, rejection, neglect, or abuse, and they affect not only how we feel but also how we think and behave.

The key distinction between emotional and physical wounds is that emotional wounds are often invisible, and because of this, they are frequently overlooked or dismissed. However, their impact can be just as severe, if not more, than physical injuries.

Common Causes of Emotional Wounds:

- **Loss or grief:** The death of a loved one, or even the loss of a significant relationship, can leave deep emotional scars.

- **Betrayal or trust violations:** Being betrayed by someone we trust can shatter our sense of security and self-worth.

- **Neglect or abandonment:** Emotional or physical neglect, particularly in childhood, can lead to feelings of unworthiness and a lack of self-confidence.

- **Abuse (physical, emotional, or sexual):** Any form of abuse can cause long-lasting psychological trauma, affecting the way we view ourselves and others.

Emotional wounds are not always the result of one-time events. They can also accumulate over time through repeated experiences, such as ongoing criticism, chronic stress, or feeling unloved. These wounds build up, shaping our perception of the world and ourselves, influencing how we navigate life.

2. The Hidden Effects of Unresolved Pain

The damage caused by emotional wounds can remain hidden for years, only surfacing in the form of negative behaviors, unhealthy coping mechanisms, and self-sabotage. People often underestimate the impact of unresolved emotional pain, but it affects nearly every aspect of life—from mental and emotional health to physical well-being and interpersonal relationships.

Mental and Emotional Impact:

- **Anxiety and depression:** Emotional wounds can lead to chronic feelings of sadness, worthlessness, and fear. Unresolved trauma can also trigger anxiety disorders and contribute to depressive symptoms.

- **Low self-esteem:** Those carrying emotional wounds may develop a negative self-image, believing they are undeserving of love, success, or happiness. This often stems from early experiences where they felt neglected, criticized, or abandoned.

- **Difficulty in trusting others:** Trust issues are common in individuals with deep emotional scars, particularly if betrayal or abandonment is part of their past. These trust issues can hinder the ability to form close, intimate relationships.

Physical Manifestations: Interestingly, unresolved emotional wounds can also manifest physically. Chronic stress, stemming from emotional pain, has been linked to a range of physical health problems, including headaches, digestive issues, weakened immune response, and even cardiovascular diseases. The mind-body connection is powerful, and when emotional pain is not addressed, it can affect the body in significant ways.

Social and Relationship Impact:

- **Attachment issues:** Unresolved emotional wounds can interfere with one's ability to form healthy attachments. Some may become overly dependent on others, seeking constant validation, while others may push people away to avoid being hurt again.

- **Repeating toxic patterns:** People with unhealed emotional wounds often find themselves repeating the same unhealthy relationship patterns, such as attracting emotionally unavailable partners or staying in toxic relationships out of fear of abandonment.

Research conducted by the American Psychological Association (APA) has found that individuals with unresolved emotional trauma are more likely to experience long-term mental health issues, including depression, anxiety, and PTSD (American Psychological Association, 2017). Furthermore, untreated emotional wounds can perpetuate a cycle of emotional instability, as they shape how we perceive and react to new experiences.

3. How Trauma Shapes Our Perceptions

Trauma has a profound effect on how we perceive the world around us. Whether it's a single traumatic event, such as an accident or a violent incident, or ongoing trauma, like prolonged emotional abuse, trauma alters the way the brain processes information and experiences. **Essentially, our brains become wired to anticipate danger, even in situations that are safe.**

Trauma and the Brain: Neuroscientific research shows that trauma significantly impacts key regions of the brain, particularly the amygdala (responsible for processing emotions and detecting threats), the hippocampus (involved in memory formation), and the prefrontal cortex (responsible for decision-making and self-regulation). **When someone experiences trauma, their brain may become**

hypervigilant, constantly scanning for signs of danger. This heightened state of alertness can make it difficult to feel safe and relaxed, even in non-threatening environments.

Shifts in Perception:

- **Negative worldview:** Individuals with emotional wounds often view the world as a dangerous place, where they are perpetually vulnerable to being hurt or betrayed. This negative worldview can lead to feelings of hopelessness and helplessness.

- **Distorted self-perception:** Emotional wounds, particularly those from early childhood, shape how we see ourselves. Traumatic experiences often lead individuals to internalize negative beliefs about their worth and capabilities. For example, a child who experienced neglect may grow up believing they are unlovable or that they don't deserve care and attention.

- **Emotional reactivity:** Trauma can make individuals more emotionally reactive to everyday situations. What may seem like a minor disagreement or criticism to others can feel overwhelming and deeply hurtful to someone with unhealed emotional wounds. This heightened emotional sensitivity can strain relationships and lead to unnecessary conflict.

Case Study: Sarah's Struggle with Trauma

Sarah's experience with emotional neglect during her childhood left her constantly seeking validation from others. As an adult, she found herself in toxic relationships, trying to "prove" her worth through pleasing others. Her trauma had shaped her perception of relationships—she believed that love was something she had to earn. Over time, Sarah realized that her pattern of seeking approval stemmed from her unresolved childhood wounds. Through therapy, she began to challenge the false beliefs about herself that had been formed by her early trauma. With time, she learned to recognize her inherent worth and to form healthier, more balanced relationships.

4. Recognizing Emotional Triggers

One of the key challenges of living with emotional wounds is dealing with triggers—situations, words, or people that evoke strong emotional reactions tied to past pain. Emotional triggers are deeply rooted in the memories of the trauma we've experienced, and when triggered, they can cause us to relive the emotional intensity of those experiences.

What Are Emotional Triggers? Emotional triggers are stimuli that set off an intense emotional response, often disproportionate to the actual situation at hand. For example, a simple argument with a partner might trigger feelings of abandonment if someone has experienced emotional neglect or betrayal in the past. Even subtle comments or gestures can serve as triggers, bringing old wounds back to the surface.

Common Emotional Triggers:

- **Rejection or abandonment:** Feelings of rejection can be intensely painful for individuals with emotional wounds related to past abandonment or betrayal.

- **Criticism or failure:** Those who experienced childhood neglect or abuse may be particularly sensitive to criticism, viewing it as confirmation of their perceived inadequacies.

- **Loss of control:** Trauma survivors often feel a strong need to be in control of their environment to prevent re-experiencing helplessness. Any loss of control can trigger feelings of anxiety or fear.

Managing Triggers: The first step in managing emotional triggers is awareness. Recognizing when and why you are triggered allows you to step back from the emotional reaction and respond more rationally. **Therapy, mindfulness practices, and journaling can help individuals identify their triggers and develop strategies to cope with them.**

Case Study: Emma's Emotional Triggers

Emma struggled with abandonment issues due to her parents' divorce during her childhood. As an adult, she found herself reacting intensely whenever her partner needed space or time apart. This triggered a deep-seated fear of abandonment, leading her to act out in ways that strained the relationship. Through counseling, Emma learned to identify this trigger and understand that her partner's need for space didn't mean he was abandoning her. With time and self-reflection, she developed healthier ways to communicate her needs without falling into old patterns of fear and insecurity.

Conclusion

Emotional wounds may be invisible, but their impact on mental, emotional, and relational health is profound. These wounds shape how we see ourselves, how we interact with others, and how we navigate life. By understanding the nature of emotional wounds and trauma, we take the first step toward healing. Recognizing the hidden effects of unresolved pain, the influence of trauma on our perceptions, and the emotional triggers that keep us trapped in old patterns allows us to begin the process of reclaiming our emotional well-being.

Healing emotional wounds is a journey—one that requires patience, self-awareness, and support. With the right tools and understanding, we can free ourselves from the grip of the past and move toward a future filled

2

THE POWER OF SELF-AWARENESS: IDENTIFYING EMOTIONAL BAGGAGE

"You can't heal what you refuse to acknowledge." –
Anonymous

Introduction

Emotional baggage is something we all carry to varying degrees. These are the unresolved feelings, traumas, and past experiences that influence our thoughts, behaviors, and relationships. While it's natural to accumulate emotional wounds over time, many of us remain unaware of the impact these hidden burdens have on our mental and emotional well-being. Without self-awareness, this emotional baggage continues to weigh us down, affecting our choices and interactions in ways that keep us stuck in cycles of pain.

In this chapter, we'll explore how self-awareness is the key to identifying and addressing emotional baggage. Through guided exercises and reflections, you will learn to recognize the unresolved issues that you may be carrying and gain insights into how they shape your present life. With self-awareness as your foundation, healing becomes not only possible but transformative.

1. Signs You're Carrying Emotional Baggage

Carrying emotional baggage can manifest in many ways, often subtly influencing your daily life. While it may not always be obvious, unresolved issues from the past tend to show up through patterns of behavior, thought processes, and emotional reactions. Becoming aware of these signs is the first step toward identifying and releasing the emotional baggage that holds you back.

Common Signs of Emotional Baggage:

- **Repeating negative patterns in relationships:**

Do you find yourself attracted to the same type of partner, only to experience similar heartbreaks? Repeated patterns in relationships, especially those marked by conflict, distrust, or emotional unavailability, often point to unresolved emotional baggage.

- **Difficulty trusting others:** If you struggle to trust people, even those close to you, it could be a sign of past betrayal or abandonment that hasn't been fully healed. This mistrust can manifest in suspicion, jealousy, or an unwillingness to open up emotionally.

- **Overreacting to minor situations:** Emotional baggage can make you hyper-sensitive to certain situations, triggering intense emotional reactions to events that seem insignificant to others. For example, a casual criticism may evoke feelings of shame or defensiveness if you've internalized negative beliefs from past experiences.

- **Fear of vulnerability:** If you find it difficult to be emotionally vulnerable, it may stem from past hurt or rejection. Avoiding vulnerability can create distance in relationships and prevent deeper connections.

- **Self-sabotage or procrastination:** Emotional baggage often creates feelings of unworthiness or fear of failure, leading to self-sabotage. **You might avoid pursuing meaningful goals or delay important decisions because deep down, unresolved emotions are holding you back.**

Exercise: Take a moment to reflect on your current life. Are there any areas where you feel stuck, frustrated, or emotionally reactive? Write down any recurring patterns in your behavior or relationships that may indicate unresolved emotional baggage. This awareness is the first step in recognizing the impact of your past.

2. Self-Reflection: Identifying the Sources of Pain

Once you've recognized the signs of emotional baggage, the next step is to trace these feelings and patterns back to their source. Emotional wounds often originate from past experiences, but the specific event or trauma may not always be immediately clear. Self-reflection can help you connect the dots between your current emotional struggles and the past events that shaped them.

Questions for Reflection:

1. **When did this pattern begin?** Think back to when you first noticed the emotional challenges or behaviors that are troubling you today. Did they emerge after a particular life event, relationship, or experience? Understanding when a pattern began can provide valuable insight into its origins.

2. **What emotions are most common in these situations?** Are you often angry, anxious, or sad in certain contexts? Identifying the emotions that frequently arise in response to specific triggers can help you pinpoint the underlying issues you need to address.

3. **How did past relationships influence your view of yourself?** Reflect on your early relationships with family, friends, or romantic partners. Did these relationships make you feel valued, safe, and supported, or did they leave you feeling unworthy, rejected, or unloved? Our sense of self is often shaped by how others treat us in our formative years.

4. **What are your greatest fears in relationships or personal pursuits?** Fears of rejection,

abandonment, or failure are often rooted in past experiences. Identifying these fears can help you understand the specific wounds that continue to affect your emotional well-being.

Case Study: Anna's Journey to Self-Awareness

Anna had always felt a deep sense of unworthiness, which affected her relationships and career. Despite being successful on the surface, she constantly doubted her abilities and felt emotionally disconnected from her partners. Through self-reflection, Anna traced her emotional baggage back to her childhood, where she had felt neglected and criticized by her parents. These early experiences had planted the belief that she wasn't good enough, and this belief continued to influence her life as an adult. By acknowledging the source of her pain, Anna was able to begin the process of healing and rebuild her self-esteem.

3. The Role of Mindfulness in Self-Awareness

Mindfulness is a powerful tool in cultivating self-awareness, particularly when it comes to identifying emotional baggage. By practicing mindfulness, you develop the ability to observe your thoughts and emotions without judgment, allowing you to gain greater insight into the patterns that control your behavior.

What is Mindfulness? Mindfulness involves paying attention to the present moment with curiosity and openness. It encourages you to focus on your thoughts, feelings, and physical sensations as they arise, without trying to change or avoid them. This practice is particularly effective in helping individuals recognize their emotional triggers and automatic reactions.

How Mindfulness Helps with Emotional Baggage:

- **Increases emotional awareness:** By tuning into your emotions as they arise, mindfulness allows you to become more aware of the feelings associated with emotional baggage. Rather than pushing painful emotions aside, mindfulness encourages you to sit with them, observe them, and understand their roots.

- **Interrupts negative thought patterns:** Emotional baggage often fuels negative self-talk and limiting beliefs. Mindfulness helps you notice these patterns as they occur, giving you the opportunity to challenge them and choose more constructive responses.

- **Reduces emotional reactivity:** When you're carrying emotional baggage, it's easy to become reactive to minor provocations. Mindfulness helps you slow down and respond thoughtfully rather than react impulsively, breaking the cycle of emotional avoidance.

Exercise: Practice mindful observation by taking five minutes each day to sit quietly and focus on your thoughts and emotions. Notice any discomfort or resistance that arises and simply observe it without judgment. Over time, this practice will help you become more attuned to the emotional baggage you're carrying and how it shows up in your daily life.

Scientific Support for Mindfulness: Research has shown that mindfulness practices can help reduce the symptoms of anxiety, depression, and emotional distress by increasing self-awareness and emotional regulation (Holzel et al., 2011). A study published in the *Journal of Clinical Psychology* found that mindfulness-based therapy led to significant improvements in individuals dealing with unresolved trauma, highlighting the power of mindfulness in healing emotional wounds (Kearney et al., 2013).

4. Breaking the Cycle of Emotional Avoidance

Avoidance is one of the most common ways people cope with emotional baggage. Rather than confronting painful emotions, many individuals choose to suppress, distract, or deny them. While avoidance may provide temporary relief, it ultimately prevents healing and perpetuates the cycle of emotional pain.

The Consequences of Emotional Avoidance:

- **Escalating emotional distress:** When you avoid dealing with your emotional baggage, the feelings don't go away—they simply get buried deeper. Over time, these unresolved emotions can intensify, leading to greater distress and emotional outbursts.

- **Physical symptoms:** Emotional avoidance can also manifest physically, contributing to chronic stress, tension headaches, digestive issues, and sleep disturbances. The body often bears the brunt of unresolved emotional pain.

- **Detachment and disconnection:** People who avoid their emotions may find it difficult to connect with others on a deep level. Emotional avoidance creates a barrier between yourself and others, leading to feelings of isolation and loneliness.

Steps to Break the Cycle:

1. **Acknowledge your emotions:** The first step to breaking the cycle of avoidance is acknowledging the emotions you've been avoiding. This can be uncomfortable at first, but it's a crucial part of the healing process.

2. **Create a safe space for emotional exploration:** Set aside time in a quiet, comfortable environment to reflect on your emotions. Journaling, meditation, or talking to a trusted friend or therapist can help you explore these feelings without judgment.

3. **Develop healthy coping mechanisms:** Instead of turning to avoidance strategies like alcohol, overeating, or distractions, learn healthier ways to cope with emotional pain. Exercise, creative expression, and mindfulness are all effective outlets for processing emotions.

Case Study: Emily's Breakthrough with Emotional Avoidance

Emily had spent years avoiding the grief and anger she felt after her parents' divorce. She buried herself in work and social activities, never allowing herself to process the pain. This emotional avoidance eventually led to burnout and emotional numbness. It wasn't until she started therapy and began practicing mindfulness that Emily confronted her emotions. By acknowledging her pain and allowing herself to grieve, she finally broke free from the emotional chains that had held her back for so long.

Conclusion

Self-awareness is the foundation of emotional healing. By identifying the emotional baggage you carry, you take the first critical step toward releasing the unresolved pain that affects your mental and emotional well-being. Through self-reflection, mindfulness, and breaking the cycle of emotional avoidance, you can begin to confront the past and free yourself from its grip.

As you continue this journey, remember that healing is a gradual process, but with each step, you'll grow stronger and more self-aware. In the next chapter, we'll explore how to cultivate self-compassion and forgiveness, two essential tools for releasing emotional baggage and embracing a more empowered life.

Resources

1. **Books:**

   - *The Power of Now* by Eckhart Tolle – A guide to living in the present moment and practicing mindfulness.

   - *Radical Acceptance* by Tara Brach – This book offers practical strategies for cultivating self-compassion and embracing all of our emotions, even the painful ones.

2. **Mindfulness Apps:**

   - Headspace

   - Calm

3. **Therapists and Counselors:** If you find it challenging to explore your emotional baggage on your own, consider seeking support from a licensed

therapist who specializes in emotional healing and trauma.

4. **Online Support Communities:** Many online forums and support groups offer a safe space for individuals to share their experiences and seek guidance on emotional healing.

3

⸺ ◆ ⸺

LETTING GO: TECHNIQUES TO RELEASE EMOTIONAL PAIN

"To let go does not mean to get rid of. To let go means to let be. When we let be with compassion, things come and go on their own." – Jack Kornfield

Introduction

Letting go of emotional pain is one of the most challenging but necessary steps in the healing journey. Emotional wounds often fester because they are carried for too long, weighing down the heart and mind. Releasing these wounds, however, is not about forgetting or dismissing the past. It is about making peace with it so that you can move forward unburdened and with a renewed sense of freedom.

This chapter will explore practical techniques that can help you release past emotional pain. From forgiveness to journaling, meditation to therapy, we'll dive into the tools you can use to let go of resentment, gain emotional clarity, and embark on a path of healing. These step-by-step strategies are designed to provide you with tangible ways to process your feelings and gradually let go of the emotional burdens that have held you back.

1. The Art of Forgiveness: Letting Go of Resentment

Forgiveness is often misunderstood. It is not about condoning or excusing harmful behavior, nor is it about reconciliation with those who have caused you pain. Instead, forgiveness is an act of liberation—a decision to let go of the resentment and anger that continues to hurt you long after the original wound was inflicted. By holding onto grudges and past hurts, we keep ourselves trapped in cycles of bitterness, which can be emotionally exhausting.

Steps to Practice Forgiveness:

1. **Acknowledge the Pain:** Before you can forgive, you must acknowledge the hurt you have experienced.

Take time to reflect on what happened, how it made you feel, and the lasting impact it has had on your emotional well-being. Ignoring or minimizing the pain will only make it harder to let go.

2. **Understand Forgiveness as a Personal Choice:** Forgiveness is not for the other person; it's for you. It is a decision to free yourself from the emotional weight of resentment. Understand that you have the power to let go, even if the person who hurt you is not sorry or has not changed.

3. **Release the Need for Justice or Retribution:** Often, we hold onto resentment because we feel that forgiving someone means letting them off the hook. However, forgiveness is not about letting the other person escape accountability; it is about releasing your need for control over their consequences. **Justice is not yours to deliver, but healing is yours to claim.**

4. **Practice Compassion:** Try to see the person who hurt you through a lens of compassion. This doesn't mean excusing their behavior, but recognizing that they, too, may have their own emotional wounds or limitations. Compassion helps you release the hold

that anger and resentment have over you.

5. **Make Forgiveness a Daily Practice:** Forgiveness is not a one-time event; it is an ongoing process. You may need to remind yourself every day of your commitment to let go of resentment. With time, the emotional charge behind the pain will diminish, and forgiveness will become more natural.

Exercise: Write a letter to the person who hurt you, expressing all of the feelings you've kept bottled up. Be as honest and open as you can. At the end of the letter, write, "I choose to forgive you, and I release you from my heart." You don't need to send the letter—this is for your emotional release.

2. Journaling for Emotional Clarity

Journaling is a powerful tool for emotional release. Writing allows you to express your deepest thoughts and feelings in a safe and private space, helping you process your emotions more clearly. **When you journal, you create a tangible record of your experiences and reflections, which can lead to insights and breakthroughs you may not have had otherwise.**

How Journaling Helps:

- **Gives you a voice:** Writing about your emotions gives them a voice, allowing you to express feelings you may have been suppressing. This can lead to a sense of relief and catharsis.

- **Clarifies your emotions:** Journaling helps you organize your thoughts and emotions, making it easier to understand the underlying causes of your pain.

- **Identifies patterns:** By regularly journaling, you can begin to notice patterns in your emotional responses, thoughts, and behaviors. This awareness is the first step toward breaking harmful cycles.

- **Promotes problem-solving:** Writing about emotional pain often leads to new perspectives and solutions. As you journal, you may uncover ways to address and resolve the pain you've been carrying.

Step-by-Step Journaling Strategy:

1. **Set aside time daily:** Dedicate at least 10-15 minutes a day to journaling. Choose a quiet space

where you won't be interrupted.

2. **Start with a prompt:** If you're unsure how to begin, use prompts like:

   - "Today, I feel..."

   - "What hurt me the most is..."

   - "What I want to let go of is..."

3. **Write freely and without judgment:** Don't worry about grammar, spelling, or structure. Let your thoughts flow naturally. The goal is to express your emotions freely.

4. **Revisit your journal:** After a week or a month, go back and read your entries. Look for recurring themes or insights that can help you better understand your emotional state.

Exercise: Try journaling specifically about forgiveness and letting go. Write about what forgiveness means to you and how you feel about the idea of releasing your emotional pain. As you journal, you may discover hidden feelings or resistance that need to be addressed.

3. Meditation and Visualization for Healing

Meditation is a powerful tool for letting go of emotional pain, as it helps you calm your mind and become more present in the moment. When combined with visualization techniques, meditation can help you process and release painful emotions, allowing you to experience a sense of peace and emotional healing.

How Meditation and Visualization Help:

- **Creates inner stillness:** Meditation quiets the mind and allows you to observe your emotions from a place of calm, rather than reacting to them. This practice helps you gain emotional distance from your pain.

- **Encourages emotional release:** Visualization techniques guide you through the process of releasing stored emotions by imagining them being physically or energetically released from your body.

- **Promotes self-compassion:** Meditation encourages self-acceptance and compassion, which are essential for emotional healing. Through meditation, you can develop a kinder and more understanding relationship with yourself.

Step-by-Step Meditation and Visualization Technique:

1. **Find a quiet space:** Sit comfortably in a quiet room where you won't be disturbed. Close your eyes and take a few deep breaths to relax your body.

2. **Focus on your breath:** Begin by focusing on your breath. Inhale deeply, hold for a few seconds, and exhale slowly. As you focus on your breathing, allow your mind to quiet down.

3. **Visualize your pain:** Once you feel calm, imagine the emotional pain you've been carrying as a physical object or dark cloud in your body. Visualize where this pain is stored—perhaps in your chest, stomach, or heart.

4. **Release the pain:** As you breathe in, imagine filling your body with healing light or warmth. As you exhale, visualize the pain leaving your body in the form of the object or cloud, dissolving into the air. With each exhale, feel the emotional burden becoming lighter.

5. **Affirm healing and release:** After a few minutes of visualization, silently repeat affirmations like:

- "I release the pain of my past."

- "I forgive and let go."

- "I am healing and at peace."

Exercise: Try this meditation and visualization technique for 10 minutes each day. With consistent practice, you will begin to feel a sense of emotional lightness and peace, as if a weight has been lifted from your heart.

4. The Role of Professional Help: Therapy and Counseling

While self-help techniques such as journaling and meditation can be effective, some emotional wounds may require deeper intervention. Therapy and counseling offer a safe and structured environment where you can work through your emotional pain with the guidance of a trained professional. Whether you're dealing with trauma, grief, or long-standing emotional wounds, therapy can provide the tools and support you need to heal.

How Therapy Helps with Emotional Release:

- **Provides a safe space for exploration:** A therapist can help you explore your emotions in a non-judgmental and confidential environment, allowing you to feel safe and supported as you confront painful experiences.

- **Offers new perspectives:** Therapists are trained to help you see your situation from different angles. They can provide insights into how your past influences your present and help you identify healthier coping mechanisms.

- **Guides you through the healing process:** Therapy often involves structured techniques like cognitive-behavioral therapy (CBT), which helps you challenge negative thought patterns and develop more constructive ways of thinking.

- **Helps with trauma and unresolved grief:** If you've experienced trauma, therapy can help you process these events in a way that allows you to heal without being overwhelmed by the pain.

Types of Therapy for Emotional Healing:

1. **Talk Therapy (Cognitive-Behavioral Therapy or CBT):**CBT helps you challenge negative thoughts and beliefs that contribute to emotional pain. This form of therapy is especially helpful for those struggling with anxiety, depression, or trauma-related issues.

2. **Trauma Therapy (EMDR or Somatic Experiencing):**EMDR (Eye Movement Desensitization and Reprocessing) and Somatic Experiencing are therapies specifically designed to help individuals process trauma and release stored emotional pain from the body.

3. **Group Therapy:** For those who feel isolated in their pain, group therapy offers the opportunity to connect with others who are going through similar experiences. Sharing your journey with others can provide validation and support.

Exercise: If you feel stuck in your healing process or overwhelmed by emotional pain, consider reaching out to a therapist. Explore different types of therapy to find what works best for you. Many therapists offer initial consultations, so you can determine if they are a good fit for your needs.

Conclusion

Letting go of emotional pain is not an overnight process, but with patience and the right tools, you can release the burdens that have weighed you down for far too long. Whether through forgiveness, journaling, meditation, or therapy, you have the power to take control of your healing journey and create emotional freedom. Each step forward brings you closer to living a life unshackled by the past, opening the door to greater peace, happiness, and self-awareness.

In the next chapter, we'll dive into the transformative power of self-compassion and how practicing kindness toward yourself can accelerate your healing process.

Resources

1. **Books:**

   - *The Body Keeps the Score* by Bessel van der Kolk – A groundbreaking book on how trauma is stored in the body and how to heal from it.

   - *Self-Compassion* by Kristin Neff – A practical

guide on how to develop self-compassion and improve emotional well-being.

2. Meditation Apps:

- Insight Timer

- Ten Percent Happier

3. Therapy Directories:

- Psychology Today (Find a Therapist)

- TherapyRoute.com

4. Support Groups:

- National Alliance on Mental Illness (NAMI) Support Groups

- Trauma Recovery Network

4

REBUILDING CONFIDENCE: FROM VULNERABILITY TO STRENGTH

"Vulnerability sounds like truth and feels like courage. Truth and courage aren't always comfortable, but they're never weakness." – Brené Brown

Introduction

Emotional healing is just the beginning of a transformative journey. Once you have started to let go of the pain from your past, the next critical step is rebuilding your confidence and sense of self-worth. Emotional wounds often leave behind scars in the form of negative beliefs, insecurity, and a fragile sense of identity. Rebuilding confidence is essential to creating a resilient mindset that allows you to thrive, not just survive.

In this chapter, we will focus on restoring your self-esteem, reshaping your beliefs about yourself, and embracing vulnerability as a source of strength. Through targeted exercises, you will learn how to break free from the limiting beliefs that have held you back and cultivate a confident, empowered self-image.

1. Reclaiming Your Self-Worth

Emotional pain often damages our sense of self-worth. We may start to believe that we are not good enough, unworthy of love, or undeserving of success. Reclaiming your self-worth after emotional healing is vital to moving forward with confidence and resilience.

How to Reclaim Your Self-Worth:

1. **Acknowledge Your Intrinsic Value:** Self-worth is not about achievements, appearance, or external validation. It's about recognizing your inherent value as a person. Reflect on the fact that you are worthy simply because you exist. Your value is not

determined by what you do or what others think of you.

2. **Challenge Negative Self-Talk:** Pay attention to the inner dialogue you have about yourself. Often, we are our own harshest critics. When negative self-talk arises—thoughts like "I'm not good enough" or "I always fail"—question their validity. Are these thoughts based on facts, or are they distorted by past emotional pain?

3. **Celebrate Your Strengths:** Take time to identify and appreciate your unique strengths and qualities. What are you proud of? What qualities have helped you overcome challenges in the past? By focusing on your strengths, you begin to rebuild a positive self-image.

4. **Set Boundaries:** Part of reclaiming self-worth is setting boundaries with others. Don't allow people to treat you in ways that undermine your confidence or self-esteem. Recognize that you deserve respect, and that means standing up for yourself and maintaining healthy boundaries.

Exercise: Write a list of five things you love about yourself—qualities, skills, or personal strengths that make you proud. Keep this list somewhere visible and read it every day as a reminder of your worth.

2. Transforming Limiting Beliefs

Limiting beliefs are self-imposed barriers that prevent us from achieving our full potential. These beliefs often stem from past experiences, trauma, or negative conditioning. If left unchallenged, they can keep you stuck in patterns of self-doubt and fear. To rebuild confidence, it's essential to identify and transform these limiting beliefs into empowering ones.

Common Limiting Beliefs and How to Overcome Them:

1. **"I'm not good enough."** This belief often develops from experiences of rejection, failure, or criticism. To challenge it, ask yourself, "What evidence do I have that I'm not good enough?" Likely, you'll find that this belief is not rooted in reality but in past emotional wounds. Replace it with an empowering affirmation like, "I am capable and deserving of

success."

2. **"I will fail if I try."** Fear of failure can hold you back from pursuing your goals and dreams. Remember that failure is not the opposite of success; it's part of the process. Every failure is a learning experience. Reframe this belief to: "I will grow and learn with each step I take."

3. **"I don't deserve love or happiness."** Emotional pain can lead to the belief that you are unworthy of love or joy. Challenge this by recognizing that everyone, including you, deserves love and happiness. Your past does not define your worth. Replace this belief with, "I am worthy of love, and I welcome happiness into my life."

Exercise to Reframe Limiting Beliefs:

1. Write down a list of limiting beliefs you hold about yourself. Be as specific as possible.

2. For each belief, ask yourself where it came from. Was it a past experience, a negative comment from someone else, or a recurring thought?

3. Now, write a new empowering belief to replace each limiting one. For example, if your limiting belief is "I'm not smart enough," reframe it to "I am constantly learning and growing."

3. Developing a Confident, Resilient Mindset

A resilient mindset is one that not only bounces back from setbacks but also learns and grows stronger from them. Confidence comes from knowing that no matter what challenges you face, you have the inner strength and resilience to overcome them.

Steps to Develop a Confident and Resilient Mindset:

1. **Embrace Growth Over Perfection: A key element of resilience is focusing on growth rather than perfection.** Mistakes and failures are inevitable, but they don't define your worth. Instead, view challenges as opportunities for learning and self-improvement.

2. **Practice Self-Compassion:** Confidence grows when you treat yourself with kindness, especially in moments of failure or struggle. Instead of beating

yourself up for not being "good enough," practice self-compassion by acknowledging your efforts and giving yourself grace.

3. **Build Emotional Grit:** Resilience requires emotional grit—the ability to stay composed in the face of adversity. Develop this by facing challenges head-on rather than avoiding them. Every time you confront a difficult situation, you build mental and emotional toughness.

4. **Focus on Your Accomplishments:** Keep track of your successes, no matter how small. Whether it's completing a project at work or having a difficult conversation, celebrate your wins. This reinforces the belief that you are capable of achieving your goals, which boosts confidence.

Exercise for Building Resilience: Write a list of three challenges you've faced in the past and how you overcame them. Reflect on the strength, skills, and determination you used to get through those difficult times. This will remind you of your resilience and ability to handle future challenges.

4. Harnessing Vulnerability as a Strength

In our culture, vulnerability is often seen as a weakness, but in reality, it is one of the greatest strengths you can cultivate. Vulnerability is the courage to be authentic and open, even when it feels uncomfortable. It allows you to form deeper connections with others and live more fully. True confidence comes from embracing your vulnerability rather than hiding it.

How Vulnerability Enhances Confidence:

1. **Increases Authenticity:** When you allow yourself to be vulnerable, you are being true to who you are. Authenticity fosters self-confidence because you no longer need to hide behind a facade. You learn to accept yourself, flaws and all.

2. **Builds Stronger Relationships:** Vulnerability creates deeper, more meaningful connections with others. When you open up and share your true feelings, you invite others to do the same, which fosters trust and strengthens relationships.

3. **Promotes Emotional Healing:** Vulnerability allows you to express your emotions freely, which is

crucial for emotional healing. When you let down your guard and acknowledge your pain, you begin to process and release it, allowing you to move forward with confidence.

4. **Fosters Courage:** It takes courage to be vulnerable, especially in a world that often equates vulnerability with weakness. By embracing vulnerability, you build emotional resilience and confidence in your ability to face life's uncertainties.

Exercise to Embrace Vulnerability: Identify an area of your life where you've been avoiding vulnerability—perhaps in your relationships, at work, or in your self-expression. Challenge yourself to take one small step toward openness. This could be having an honest conversation with a loved one, sharing your thoughts in a group setting, or expressing your true feelings about something important to you.

Conclusion

Rebuilding confidence after emotional healing is about more than just feeling good about yourself—it's about reclaiming your power, reframing limiting beliefs, and recognizing that vulnerability is a strength, not a weakness. As you work through these exercises, remember that confidence is not built overnight. It's a journey of self-discovery, healing, and personal growth.

In the next chapter, we will explore how to create new, empowering narratives for your life and shape a future defined by strength, resilience, and emotional freedom.

Resources

1. **Books:**

   - *The Gifts of Imperfection* by Brené Brown – A guide to embracing vulnerability and cultivating self-worth.

   - *Mindset: The New Psychology of Success* by Carol S. Dweck – A book that explores the power of a growth mindset.

2. **Workshops and Courses:**

   - *The Power of Vulnerability* (Brené Brown's course on courage and vulnerability).

3. **Support Groups:**

   - Confidence-building workshops or self-esteem support groups in your area.

4. Online Resources:

- ○ TED Talks: *The Power of Vulnerability* by Brené Brown.

4. **Online Resources:**

- ○ TED Talks: *The Power of Vulnerability* by Brené Brown.

5

BUILDING EMOTIONAL RESILIENCE FOR FUTURE CHALLENGES

"Resilience is not just about bouncing back; it's about bouncing forward." – Christine Caine

Introduction

Emotional resilience is the ability to adapt and recover from life's challenges, setbacks, and emotional wounds. It is the mental reservoir of strength that helps you cope with stress, adversity, and trauma. Building emotional resilience is essential for maintaining your progress after healing from past wounds. It empowers you to face future challenges with confidence and strength, preventing old wounds from reopening and disrupting your journey.

In this chapter, we will explore what emotional resilience is, how to establish strong emotional boundaries, effective stress management techniques, and daily habits that fortify resilience. By equipping yourself with these tools, you can cultivate a robust emotional foundation that supports your growth and well-being.

1. What is Emotional Resilience?

Emotional resilience is the capacity to recover quickly from difficulties. It involves maintaining a positive outlook, adapting to change, and managing stress in healthy ways. Resilient individuals tend to have a growth mindset, viewing challenges as opportunities for learning rather than insurmountable obstacles.

Key Components of Emotional Resilience:

- **Self-awareness:** Understanding your emotions, triggers, and responses.

- **Emotional regulation:** The ability to manage and respond to your emotions appropriately.

- **Adaptability:** Being flexible in the face of change and uncertainty.

- **Support systems:** Relying on relationships and networks for emotional support.

- **Purpose and goals:** Having a clear sense of purpose helps you stay motivated through challenges.

Research Insight: A study published in the *Journal of Happiness Studies* found that individuals with higher emotional resilience tend to experience lower levels of stress and anxiety, leading to better overall mental health outcomes.

2. How to Develop Stronger Emotional Boundaries

Emotional boundaries define what you are comfortable with in relationships, protecting your emotional space from being compromised. Establishing strong boundaries is a crucial step in building resilience, as it prevents emotional burnout and ensures you prioritize your well-being.

Strategies for Developing Emotional Boundaries:

1. **Identify Your Limits:** Reflect on your emotional triggers and stressors. What situations, people, or activities drain your energy? Knowing your limits helps you recognize when boundaries need to be set.

2. **Communicate Clearly:** Once you understand your limits, communicate them to others. Use "I" statements to express your needs and feelings without placing blame. For example, "I feel overwhelmed when I take on too many responsibilities. I need to say no to additional tasks right now."

3. **Learn to Say No:** Saying no is a vital skill in boundary-setting. Practice asserting your right to decline requests that feel overwhelming or are not aligned with your priorities.

4. **Assess Your Relationships:** Evaluate the people in your life and how they affect your emotional well-being. Surround yourself with individuals who respect your boundaries and support your healing journey.

Exercise for Boundary-Setting: Write down three situations where you feel your boundaries are frequently crossed. Next to each situation, identify what boundaries you need to establish. Finally, practice expressing these boundaries in a calm and assertive manner.

3. Managing Stress and Anxiety During Healing

Stress and anxiety can significantly impact your emotional resilience and overall well-being, especially during the healing process. It's essential to develop effective strategies for managing these feelings to maintain emotional balance.

Effective Stress Management Techniques:

1. **Mindfulness and Meditation:** Practicing mindfulness and meditation helps ground you in the present moment, reducing anxiety and stress. Regular mindfulness practices can improve emotional regulation and resilience.

2. **Physical Activity:** Engaging in regular physical activity releases endorphins, which are natural stress relievers. Exercise can boost your mood, improve your health, and provide an outlet for pent-up emotions.

3. **Deep Breathing Exercises:** Deep breathing can activate your body's relaxation response, helping to lower stress levels. Practice inhaling deeply through your nose, holding for a few seconds, and exhaling slowly through your mouth.

4. **Journaling:** Writing about your thoughts and feelings can be therapeutic. It allows you to process emotions and clarify your thoughts, reducing anxiety and stress levels.

Research Insight: A study in *Psychological Bulletin* highlighted that mindfulness practices significantly reduce stress and anxiety levels, leading to enhanced emotional resilience and well-being.

Exercise: Set aside 10 minutes daily for mindfulness practice or deep breathing exercises. Find a quiet space, close your eyes, and focus on your breath. Notice any sensations or thoughts that arise without judgment.

4. Daily Habits to Fortify Emotional Resilience

Building emotional resilience is an ongoing process that requires consistent practice and commitment. Developing daily habits can significantly enhance your emotional well-being and prepare you for future challenges.

Daily Habits for Resilience:

1. **Gratitude Practice:** Cultivating gratitude shifts your focus from negative experiences to positive aspects of your life. Each day, write down three things you are grateful for. This simple practice can boost your mood and overall outlook.

2. **Positive Affirmations:** Incorporate positive affirmations into your daily routine to counter negative self-talk and build self-esteem. Choose affirmations that resonate with you and repeat them regularly.

3. **Connect with Others:** Maintain social connections with supportive friends and family. Engage in regular conversations, share experiences, and seek support when needed. Social connections are a vital aspect of emotional resilience.

4. **Limit Exposure to Negativity:** Be mindful of your media consumption, including news and social media. Constant exposure to negative information

can heighten stress and anxiety. Curate your media intake to include uplifting and positive content.

Exercise for Building Daily Resilience Habits: Create a "resilience routine" that incorporates at least three of the habits mentioned above. Dedicate a specific time each day for this routine, making it a non-negotiable part of your self-care.

Conclusion

Building emotional resilience is a vital step in safeguarding your mental and emotional well-being. By understanding emotional resilience, establishing strong boundaries, effectively managing stress, and incorporating daily resilience-building habits, you lay a solid foundation for facing future challenges with confidence.

As you cultivate emotional resilience, remember that setbacks are a natural part of life. Resilience does not mean you will never face difficulties; rather, it equips you with the tools and mindset to navigate those challenges effectively. In the next chapter, we will explore the power of gratitude and its role in fostering emotional well-being and resilience.

Resources

1. **Books:**

   - *Resilience: The Science of Mastering Life's Greatest Challenges* by Steven M. Southwick and Dennis S. Charney – An insightful book exploring the science behind resilience.

   - *The Resilience Factor* by Karen Reivich and Andrew Shatté – A practical guide on building resilience through cognitive and emotional skills.

2. **Online Courses:**

   - Coursera: Resilience Skills in a Time of Uncertainty

   - Udemy: Building Resilience: A Practical Guide

3. **Apps:**

   - Headspace – A meditation app that provides resources for mindfulness and stress management.

   - Calm – An app focusing on meditation, sleep,

and relaxation techniques.

4. Support Groups:

- Mental Health America (MHA) – Offers resources and support for individuals seeking emotional resilience and well-being.

6

———— ◆ ————

TURNING TRAUMA INTO YOUR GREATEST STRENGTH

"The wound is the place where the Light enters you." – Rumi

Introduction

Trauma can feel like an insurmountable obstacle, casting a long shadow over your life and choices. Yet, with the right perspective, these emotional wounds can become the very foundation of your strength and growth. This chapter will guide you through the process of reframing your past trauma into a source of resilience and empowerment.

We'll explore how to transform your pain into purpose, share success stories that illustrate the power of healing, and encourage you to embrace your healed self with pride and intention. Ultimately, your journey can serve as a beacon of hope for others navigating their own paths of healing.

1. Transforming Pain into Purpose

The first step in turning trauma into strength is recognizing that your pain can inform your purpose. Many individuals who have experienced trauma find that their struggles ultimately lead them to a deeper understanding of themselves and their values. This transformation can ignite a passion for helping others, advocating for change, or pursuing personal growth.

Steps to Transform Pain into Purpose:

- **Reflect on Your Experience:** Take time to journal or meditate on your trauma. What lessons have you learned? How has your perspective shifted? Acknowledging the impact of your experience is crucial for reframing it.

- **Identify Your Passion:** Consider how your experience has shaped your interests. Do you feel drawn to mental health advocacy, creative expression, or community service? Identifying a passion linked to your experience can provide direction and motivation.

- **Set Meaningful Goals:** Create specific, achievable goals that align with your newfound purpose. These goals will help channel your energy and determination into constructive action, turning your pain into a source of inspiration for yourself and others.

Case Study: Emily's Journey

Emily, a survivor of childhood trauma, realized that her experiences fueled her desire to help others facing similar challenges. After years of therapy and self-discovery, she became a mental health advocate, sharing her story through workshops and social media. Emily's pain transformed into purpose, inspiring countless individuals to seek help and find hope.

2. Success Stories of Strength After Trauma

The path to healing is often paved with stories of resilience and triumph. Understanding that you are not alone in your journey can empower you to embrace your strength. Here, we share a few inspiring success stories that exemplify the transformative power of healing.

Case Study: Jessica's Triumph

Jessica experienced a traumatic event in her early twenties that left her feeling lost and disconnected. After seeking therapy and engaging in self-care practices, she began writing a memoir about her journey. Her book, which chronicles her struggles and healing, became a bestseller, giving her a platform to speak about trauma and recovery. Today, Jessica conducts workshops that empower others to reclaim their narratives and find strength in their stories.

Case Study: Maria's Advocacy

After surviving an abusive relationship, Maria dedicated her life to advocating for domestic violence survivors. She founded a nonprofit organization that provides resources, support, and education for those affected by abuse. Maria's story showcases how one person's healing journey can spark change and help countless others find their voices.

Research Insight: Studies indicate that sharing personal experiences of trauma can lead to improved mental health outcomes. A review published in *The Journal of*

Trauma & Dissociation highlights the therapeutic benefits of storytelling, illustrating how it can promote healing and connection with others.

3. Living Empowered: Building a Future of Peace and Confidence

Once you have reframed your trauma and seen it as a source of strength, the next step is to embrace your empowered self and build a future rooted in peace and confidence. This transformation involves embracing new habits, setting boundaries, and surrounding yourself with supportive people.

Strategies for Living Empowered:

- **Practice Self-Compassion:** Recognize that healing is a journey filled with ups and downs. Treat yourself with kindness and understanding, just as you would for a friend.

- **Surround Yourself with Positivity:** Build a supportive network of friends, family, and mentors who uplift you. Engage with people who inspire you to grow and thrive.

- **Set Healthy Boundaries:** Establish boundaries that protect your emotional well-being. Be intentional about the relationships and environments you engage with, ensuring they align with your values and support your growth.

- **Focus on Personal Growth:** Commit to lifelong learning and self-improvement. Explore new interests, take courses, or pursue hobbies that nourish your spirit and promote confidence.

Exercise: Create a vision board that represents your empowered self. Include images, quotes, and symbols that resonate with your journey and aspirations. Place it in a space where you will see it daily, serving as a reminder of your strength and the future you are building.

4. Using Your Story to Inspire and Empower Others

Your journey of healing and transformation can be a powerful tool for inspiring others. By sharing your story, you not only validate your experience but also create a sense of community for those who may be struggling.

Ways to Share Your Story:

- **Public Speaking:** Consider speaking at local events, schools, or community organizations. Sharing your story in person can have a profound impact on those in attendance.

- **Writing:** Write articles, blog posts, or even a book detailing your journey. Sharing your experiences in written form can reach a broader audience and provide resources for those in need.

- **Social Media:** Use platforms like Instagram, Twitter, or Facebook to share your story and connect with others. Social media can be a powerful tool for advocacy and community building.

- **Mentorship:** Offer your support to others who may be on a similar healing journey. Sharing your insights and guidance can help empower those navigating their paths.

Research Insight: According to a study in *Psychological Science*, sharing personal narratives can foster social connection and increase feelings of belonging among individuals, making it a valuable tool for healing both for the storyteller and the audience.

Conclusion

Turning trauma into strength is a deeply personal journey that requires courage, vulnerability, and determination. By reframing your experiences, embracing your healed self, and using your story to empower others, you can transform pain into purpose and inspire change.

As you move forward, remember that your journey is unique, and your story holds the potential to make a profound impact. Embrace your power, honor your healing, and step boldly into a future filled with peace and confidence. The next chapter will explore the ongoing process of healing, emphasizing the importance of continuous growth and self-discovery.

Resources

1. **Books:**

   - *The Body Keeps the Score* by Bessel van der Kolk – A comprehensive guide to understanding trauma and its effects on the body and mind.

- *Rising Strong* by Brené Brown – An exploration of vulnerability and the power of storytelling in overcoming adversity.

2. **Support Groups:**

- National Alliance on Mental Illness (NAMI) – Offers support and resources for individuals experiencing mental health challenges, including trauma.

- Trauma Recovery Network – Provides support and resources for survivors of trauma.

3. **Online Platforms:**

- Meetup.com – Find local groups focused on healing, self-improvement, and sharing experiences.

- Instagram and Twitter – Follow mental health advocates and organizations to connect with others sharing their healing journeys.

4. **Workshops and Retreats:**

- Look for local workshops or retreats focused on healing, personal growth, and resilience-building.

Engaging in these experiences can deepen your understanding and provide valuable tools for your journey.

Conclusion: Moving Forward with Confidence and Peace

"The only way out is through." – Robert Frost

As we reach the conclusion of this journey through healing and emotional growth, it's important to reflect on the key insights we've explored together. Healing is not a destination but a continual process—a transformative journey that empowers you to embrace life with confidence and peace. This chapter will summarize the core messages of our exploration and motivate you to carry these lessons forward, encouraging you to practice self-awareness, self-love, and resilience as you step into your new life.

1. The Power of Healing: A New Beginning

Healing is a profound act of self-love that creates space for new beginnings. It allows you to confront and release the emotional wounds that have held you captive, providing the opportunity to redefine your narrative. Recognizing the power of healing means understanding that your past does not define you; instead, it informs your present and shapes your future.

Key Takeaways:

- **Acknowledge Your Journey:** Every step you've taken to heal is an important part of your story. Acknowledge the progress you've made, no matter how small it may seem.

- **Embrace Change:** Healing encourages personal growth, inviting you to explore new paths and opportunities. Be open to the changes that come with this journey.

- **Cultivate Hope:** Healing can ignite a sense of hope that propels you forward. Embrace this hope as you visualize your future filled with possibility.

Reflecting on these takeaways can serve as a powerful reminder of the transformative power of your healing journey. Embrace this new beginning as a chance to build the life you desire—one rooted in love, compassion, and resilience.

2. Sustaining Peace and Confidence in Everyday Life

As you move forward, sustaining the peace and confidence you've cultivated during your healing process is essential. Here are some strategies to integrate into your daily life:

Daily Practices:

- **Self-Care Rituals:** Prioritize self-care activities that nurture your mind, body, and spirit. Whether it's meditation, exercise, or creative expression, these rituals can reinforce your sense of well-being.

- **Mindfulness:** Incorporate mindfulness practices into your routine. Staying present can help you manage stress, reduce anxiety, and maintain a balanced perspective.

- **Gratitude Journaling:** Keep a gratitude journal to remind yourself of the positive aspects of your life. Regularly reflecting on what you're thankful for can foster a positive mindset and reinforce feelings of self-worth.

- **Community Engagement:** Surround yourself with supportive people who uplift and inspire you. Engaging with a community that shares your values can create a sense of belonging and reinforce your commitment to healing.

Implementing these practices can help you sustain the peace and confidence you've gained, allowing you to navigate life's challenges with grace and resilience.

3. Living Free from the Past

Ultimately, the goal of healing is to live free from the burdens of the past. This freedom allows you to embrace each day with a renewed sense of purpose and joy. By letting go of old patterns and beliefs that no longer serve you, you create space for growth and fulfillment.

Strategies for Living Free:

- **Reframe Your Story:** Continuously work on reframing your narrative. Instead of viewing your past as a limitation, see it as a testament to your strength and resilience.

- **Set Healthy Boundaries:** Protect your energy by

establishing boundaries with people and situations that may trigger past wounds. This practice will empower you to maintain your emotional well-being.

- **Celebrate Your Achievements:** Regularly acknowledge and celebrate your successes, both big and small. This practice reinforces your self-worth and motivates you to continue striving for personal growth.

By consciously choosing to live free from the past, you open the door to a future filled with possibilities. This commitment to yourself reflects your dedication to a life of peace, confidence, and resilience.

Final Thoughts

As you conclude this journey of healing, remember that the road ahead is one of continuous growth and exploration. Embrace the lessons learned, carry forward the strategies that resonate with you, and be gentle with yourself as you navigate life's ups and downs.

You have the power to create a future that is not only defined by your past but enriched by the strength and wisdom gained from your experiences. As you step into this new chapter, may you do so with confidence, peace, and an unwavering belief in your ability to heal and thrive.

Resources for Continued Growth

1. **Books:**

   - *You Are Here: An Owner's Manual for Dangerous Minds* by Jenny Lawson – A humorous yet profound exploration of mental health and self-acceptance.

   - *Radical Acceptance* by Tara Brach – A guide to embracing yourself and your life through mindfulness and compassion.

2. **Support Groups:**

   - Online forums and local support groups for those healing from trauma. Websites like Psychology Today can help you find groups in your area.

3. **Podcasts:**

   - *Unlocking Us* by Brené Brown – Conversations about vulnerability, courage, and what it means to be human.

- *Therapy Chat* – Discussions on trauma-informed therapy and emotional wellness.

4. **Online Resources:**

- Mental Health America (MHA) – Provides resources, tools, and support for individuals navigating their mental health journeys.

Embrace your journey of healing with courage and an open heart. Your past is part of your story, but it does not define your future. Here's to a life filled with peace, confidence, and endless possibilities!

May I Ask You For A Small Favor?

I want to express my sincere gratitude for choosing to invest your time in reading this book. Your decision to explore this work among countless others means a lot to me.

I hope that within these pages, you've discovered actionable insights that can enhance your daily life. Your journey doesn't have to end here, though.

May I kindly request an additional 30 seconds of your valuable time?

Sharing your thoughts about the book through a review would be immensely appreciated. Your review serves as a beacon, guiding other readers to take a chance on my books. It's a small gesture that carries significant weight in the world of authors.

To submit your review effortlessly, please click on the link below. It will take you directly to the book's review page:

"Heal Your Past"

Alternatively, you can also find the "**Reviews Section**" of this book's page on Amazon.

Your review will require just a minute of your time, but will make a monumental difference in helping me connect with a broader audience and I eagerly look forward to reading your review.

Once again, thank you for your unwavering support of my work.

DISCLAIMER

This book is for educational purposes only. Readers acknowledge the author does not render legal, financial, medical, or professional advice. The content within this book has been derived from various sources. Please consult a licensed professional before attempting any techniques outlined in this book.

By reading this document, the reader agrees that under no circumstances is the author responsible for any direct or indirect losses incurred as a result of the use of the information contained within this document, including but not limited to errors, omissions, or inaccuracies.

Adherence to all applicable laws and regulations, including international, federal, state, and local governing professional licensing, business practices, advertising, and all other jurisdictions, is the sole responsibility of the purchaser or reader.

Neither the author nor the publisher assumes any responsibility or liability whatsoever on behalf of the purchaser or reader of these materials. Any perceived slight of any individual or organization is purely unintentional.